Beginner's Guide to
LOW CARB

OVERCOME DIET OVERWHELM WITH
PRACTICAL INSIGHTS AND STRATEGIES FOR
INCREASED ENERGY, BETTER BLOOD SUGAR CONTROL,
AND WEIGHT LOSS WITHOUT HUNGER

RIKKE B. ESKILDSEN

TABLE OF CONTENTS

FOREWORD

WHAT CAN YOU EXPECT FROM THIS BOOK?

The purpose of this book is to guide you – as a beginner – through the basic principles and practices of a Low Carb diet. I aim to make the transition to a Low Carb lifestyle as simple and straightforward as possible, while providing you with the necessary tools and knowledge to achieve your health and weight loss goals.

SIMPLE AND PRACTICAL ADVICE

This book is not intended as a cookbook (although you will find suggestions for a weekly meal plan with accompanying recipes at the end of the book), but as a practical guide with easy strategies and tips for changing your lifestyle. It is designed to be a practical guide that helps you understand what a Low Carb diet entails, and how you can easily implement it in your daily life. I delve into the various foods you should include and avoid, as well as how to keep it simple and practical, so your journey towards a healthier lifestyle becomes as smooth as possible.

I hope that with this book, you will experience how weight loss can actually be achieved without starvation diets and boring food.

Happy reading.

Best regards,
Rikke

INTRODUCTION

I had tried almost everything

I want to start by sharing my own story and explaining how, after many years, I finally understood the connection between our blood sugar and our weight. Most importantly, I want to inspire you on how you can also get started and achieve success in your own weight loss journey with the help of a Low Carb diet.

As a child, I was always active and slim, but as time went on, the pounds began to creep up on me. During business school, there were parties and boyfriends, and eventually, I indulged a bit too much in all the fun.

Later, when I got an apprenticeship as a graphic designer – a rather sedentary job – and drove to and from work every day, my lunch was often bought from the local grocery store. Some days, it was followed by a bag of candy for dessert. Gradually, the number on the scale started to increase, and I began looking for ways to lose weight.

IN THE BEGINNING IT WAS EASY

The first diets went quite well. I ate whole grains and low-fat foods and quickly lost some pounds... but it was a short-lived success, and I regained all the weight... plus more!

After that, I tried soup diets, powder diets, diet pills, and weight loss clubs – along with extra exercise – but nothing helped. I became more and more unhappy and felt like a huge failure! I was always on a diet, always hungry and tired, and I felt more and more unsuccessful.

I thought it was my own fault, since I couldn't succeed and kept falling off the wagon. It became increasingly embarrassing that I couldn't stick to it.

SWEDISH DOCTORS HELPED THEIR PATIENTS LOSE WEIGHT

One day, I talked to my mother, who has also struggled with being overweight for a large part of her life and subsequently also with type 2 diabetes. She had heard that Swedish doctors had found a way to help people with diabetes and overweight – and they had great success.

I started reading a lot on the internet, watched many videos, and bought and read numerous books. Most of my waking hours were now spent seeking new knowledge, and suddenly the pieces began to fall into place.

I could suddenly understand the vicious cycle I had entered, and it now made sense why I couldn't succeed, but instead kept gaining weight.

FINALLY, THE WEIGHT BEGAN TO DROP

The common thread in all the new knowledge I had gained was that if you are overweight, you need to cut down on carbohydrates. I began to implement the simple principles in my diet and could now feel how I started to lose weight without hunger and difficulty.

At the same time, I could follow my mother on the sidelines, who also began to lose weight for the first time in many years – and even better – I could see how she gradually reduced her diabetes medication.

WEIGHT LOSS IS NOT JUST ABOUT CALORIES

I have gained a greater understanding of how the body works, and how it is affected by the food we eat.
I now know that weight loss is not "just" about eating fewer calories than you burn, and that you shouldn't just

exercise a lot and eat whole grains and low-fat foods. It simply doesn't work for everyone.

I have learned about the key that allows you to lose weight while eating good and satisfying food – and it is this experience and knowledge that I want to share with you, so that you also can succeed with your weight loss.

So...

If you have followed the common dietary advice to eat less and exercise more without success, don't give up – you can also shed those unwanted pounds (without yet another starvation diet) and gain more energy and joy.

Chapter One

WHAT IS LOW CARB?

Low Carb, or low-carbohydrate, is a dietary strategy that involves reducing the intake of carbohydrates and increasing the intake of proteins and healthy fats. Carbohydrates are one of the three macronutrients, along with proteins and fats, that our bodies use for energy.

When you follow a Low Carb diet, limiting your carbohydrate intake to a minimum helps stabilize your blood sugar levels. This is because the body produces less insulin – a hormone that regulates blood sugar and promotes fat storage – due to the reduced carbohydrate consumption.

One of the primary reasons people choose a Low Carb diet is its effectiveness in weight loss. When the body does not receive enough carbohydrates to burn for energy, it begins to burn fat reserves instead, leading to weight loss.

In addition to weight loss, many people who follow a Low Carb diet experience a range of health benefits, including increased energy levels, improved mental focus, and stabilized blood sugar levels. It can also help reduce the risk of chronic diseases such as type 2 diabetes, heart disease, and certain types of cancer (source: https://www. dietdoctor.com/low-carb/benefits).

A Low Carb diet does not have to be complicated. It is about choosing the right foods, such as vegetables, meat, fish, eggs, nuts, and healthy fats, while avoiding sugar, starch, and processed foods. By focusing on whole and natural foods, you can enjoy delicious and satisfying meals that help you achieve your health and weight loss goals.

Low Carb eating is not about depriving yourself of tasty food, but about making better choices for your health and well-being. By understanding and implementing the principles of a Low Carb lifestyle, you can take control of your diet, and begin the journey towards a healthier and more energized life.

I will explain it further during the different chapters in the book.

Chapter Two

SUGAR – THE REAL VILLAIN?

I want to start by looking at the sugar hidden in our food – what happens when you eat it, and why it can make it difficult for you to lose weight.

Most people are now aware that consuming too much sugar is not healthy for the body... but how much is "too much sugar" exactly?

Adults usually have the equivalent of about 1 teaspoon of sugar circulating in their blood at all times. If more sugar enters the bloodstream than this, the body releases the hormone insulin, which acts to "clean up" and return our blood sugar levels to normal.

In short, insulin ensures that the sugar we consume is transported into our cells and muscles, so we can use it as energy now if needed, or later if tougher times come... those tougher times rarely come nowadays, as a big part of us have constant access to food.

The challenge is that our cells and muscles have limited capacity – and when they are full, the liver converts the excess sugar into fat... and unlike our cells and muscles, our "fat storage" unfortunately has no limits – we can store as much fat as possible!

When we consume large amounts of carbohydrates at once, our blood sugar spikes quickly, and the pancreas produces a large amount of insulin, causing our blood sugar to drop rapidly again.

When this happens, we often become hungry again quickly, starting a vicious cycle... we eat more frequently than needed, while the hormone insulin is activated.

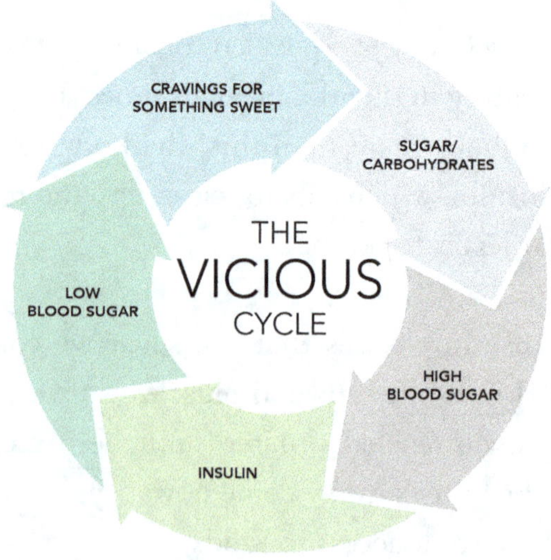

When we fill our carbohydrate stores, we have immediate energy for between 12 to 24 hours. This means that if we eat a lot of sugar and/or carbohydrates, before our stores are empty, the body has to store the excess energy as fat, as it can't put it anywhere else.

Since most people eat at least three times a day, the body rarely has the chance to empty its carbohydrate stores, and insulin is therefore often active to "store fat"... and this is, in short, how we gain weight.

To burn our stored fat, we need to avoid having too much excess sugar in the blood – so the hormone insulin does not constantly instruct the body to store the excess sugar as fat.

Cutting down on sugar in the form of candy, soda, and cake is a good start, but there are many other foods that also affect our blood sugar – and I will look at those here.

Foods like bread, rice, potatoes, pasta, chips, muesli, juice, etc., contain a lot of carbohydrates/starch – and these are all broken down into sugars in our intestines. These sugars are absorbed into our blood, raising our blood sugar level... and this is something we should avoid, so insulin doesn't come into play and "store fat."

On the following pages, you can see some examples of how much our blood sugar is affected by certain foods... and remember that the body only needs 1 teaspoon of sugar in the blood at all times...

HOW THESE FOODS AFFECT YOUR BLOOD SUGAR

Dr. David Unwin is an award-winning general practitioner from England, and he has developed these charts that are now used to help people with overweight and diabetes.

The following charts show how selected foods affect our blood sugar compared to consuming a certain number of teaspoons of sugar (4 grams each).
Source: www.phcuk.org/sugar

Food Item	Serving	Affect on Blood Sugar (compared with one 4g teaspoon of table sugar)
Banana	120 gr.	5,9
Grapes (dark)	120 gr.	4,0
Apple	120 gr.	2,2
Watermelon	120 gr.	1,8
Nectarines	120 gr.	1,5
Strawberries	120 gr.	1,4

Food Item	Serving	Affect on Blood Sugar (compared with one 4g teaspoon of table sugar)
Basmati Rice	150 gr.	**10,1**
Potato (white, boiled)	150 gr.	**9,1**
French Fries	150 gr.	**7,5**
Spaghetti (boiled)	180 gr.	**6,6**

Food Item	Serving	Affect on Blood Sugar (compared with one 4g teaspoon of table sugar)
White Bread	30 gr.	**3,7**
Wholemeal	30 gr.	**3,0**
Pita (wholemeal)	30 gr.	**2,9**

Food Item	Serving	Affect on Blood Sugar (compared with one 4g teaspoon of table sugar)
Cornflakes	30 gr.	**8,4**
Coco Pops	30 gr.	**7,3**
Bran Flakes	30 gr.	**4,8**
Special K	30 gr.	**4,0**
Oat Porrige	30 gr.	**3,3**

Food Item	Serving	Affect on Blood Sugar (compared with one 4g teaspoon of table sugar)
Pure Apple Juice	2 dl.	**8,6**
Sweet Corn (boiled)	80 gr.	**4,0**
Broccoli	80 gr.	**0,2**
Eggs	60 gr.	**0,0**

Other good foods that do not affect blood sugar could, for example, be various meats, chicken, fatty fish, butter, oil, cabbage, mushrooms, cheese and almonds

Example of a traditional "healthy" breakfast:

Food Item	Serving	Affect on Blood Sugar (compared with one 4g teaspoon of table sugar)	
Bran Flakes	30 gr.	3,7	
Milk	1,25 dl.	1,0	
Brown Toast	30 gr.	3,0	
Pure Apple Juice	2 dl.	8,6	
Total for this breakfast: 16.3 teaspoons			

The above example of a traditional "healthy" breakfast would impact your blood sugar the same as if you ate 16.3 teaspoons of sugar!

Scan the QR-code to download printable charts.

AVOID ACTIVATING THE HORMONE INSULIN TOO OFTEN IF YOU WANT TO LOSE WEIGHT

As you can see, sugar hides in many different places – and maybe also in places you hadn't thought of...

So if you want to lose weight, it is important that you don't consume more sugar than your body needs (approximately 1 teaspoon at all times). If you do, you activate the hormone insulin, which ensures that the excess sugar is converted into fat.

> The more normal your insulin level is, the greater the chance you have to get rid of your fat stores.

I hope you have become more curious about how much sugar the food you eat actually contains... and also about the role of insulin in relation to weight loss.

Our insulin level is the key to whether we gain or lose weight – and unfortunately, many people are unaware of this crucial detail. I want to change that, so that weight loss can become an easier task – and this is where the Low Carb diet comes into play – so let's roll up our sleeves and get started.

Chapter Three

WHAT'S IN YOUR KITCHEN CABINETS?

If you're the type to keep a stash of candy and cakes, and you find it hard to resist them, I recommend clearing them out, or having someone hide them for you. It can be difficult to stick to good intentions, if there are always tempting treats within reach.

When you decide to switch to a Low Carb diet, it's important to start with a solid foundation – and that begins in your kitchen. By ensuring your kitchen cabinets are stocked with the right foods, you can make the transition to a Low Carb lifestyle much easier. Let's start by taking a look at what's in your kitchen cabinets, and how you can optimize your kitchen for success.

CLEAN OUT YOUR KITCHEN CABINETS

The first step towards a Low Carb lifestyle is to clean out your kitchen cabinets. Take everything out, and lay it on the kitchen counter, so you can see what you have. Go through each item and determine if it fits into a Low Carb diet. Here are some things you should consider removing:

SUGAR AND SUGAR SUBSTITUTES

Sugar is one of the biggest culprits, when it comes to high carbohydrate intake and negative health effects. It can be found in many forms, not just obvious sweets and desserts, but also in many processed foods. Here are some sugar sources to avoid:

- **Sugar:** White sugar, brown sugar, cane sugar, and other forms of refined sugar.
- **Sugary drinks:** Soda, sports drinks, energy drinks, and sugary juice products.
- **Sugary foods:** Cakes, cookies, candy, ice cream, and other desserts.
- **Hidden sugar:** Many processed foods such as ketchup, salad dressings, marinades, deli meats, and ready meals can contain hidden sugars.

GRAINS AND STARCHES

Grains and starches are high in carbohydrates, and can cause large fluctuations in blood sugar levels. By avoiding or minimizing these foods, you can better control your blood sugar and promote desired weight loss. Here are examples of some grain- and starch-based foods to avoid:

- **Wheat-based products:** Bread, pasta, cakes, cookies, and other baked goods.
- **Rice:** White rice, brown rice, and other rice-based products.
- **Potatoes:** Regular potatoes, sweet potatoes, potato chips, and fries.
- **Corn:** Corn, cornmeal, cornstarch, and popcorn.

PROCESSED FOODS AND HIDDEN CARBOHYDRATES

Processed foods are often filled with hidden carbohydrates, unhealthy fats, and additives that can be detrimental to your health and weight loss goals.

These foods are often highly processed, and can contain many hidden ingredients. Here are some processed foods to avoid:

- **Processed snacks:** Chips, crackers, snack bars, and pre-packaged cakes.
- **Ready meals:** Frozen meals, canned soups, and ready meals, that often contain many additives and hidden carbohydrates.

- **Sugary sauces and dressings:** Many sauces, salad dressings, and marinades contain hidden sugars and other carbohydrates.

In the 1980s, the fear of natural fat took hold, and light products appeared everywhere. When you eat less fat, you eat more carbohydrates to feel full. This is where the worst obesity and diabetes epidemic in history took off. It hit the USA hardest – the homeland of fat phobia. But even in Scandinavia, the proportion of overweight people has increased dramatically since 1989. Today we know that the fear of real food with normal fat content was a mistake.

DietDoctor

----

Chapter Four

2 STRATEGIES FOR WEIGHT LOSS

As you may have discovered by now, many of the foods we thought were so healthy may not be quite as healthy after all… at least not in the quantities consumed daily by many. Carbohydrates are the part of our diet that raise our blood sugar, causing the hormone insulin to increase and putting the body into "storage mode."

"So, can I never eat carbohydrates again?"

Of course, you can, but if you want to shed those extra pounds, you need to limit them for a period.

Since we are all different, I will present two different strategies that you can try, if you want to cut down on your carbohydrates.

STRATEGY #1: COUNT YOUR CARBS

If you are the type who finds it okay to weigh your food

and keep track of your intake, for example, via an app on your phone, then by all means continue doing so. Instead of monitoring your calories,

I recommend focusing on your carbohydrates instead. Try aiming for 20-50 grams of carbohydrates per day and don't worry about your calorie count – that will be a good place to start. If you can get close to 20 grams of carbohydrates per day, it will give you the best result.

STRATEGY #2: MAX 5 GRAMS OF CARBS PER 100 GRAMS

If you are not keen on measuring and weighing, you can try starting with this simple method: choose foods that have a maximum of 5 grams of carbohydrates per 100 grams. If you choose this strategy, you will automatically keep your carbohydrate intake at a good level without having to count and weigh your food.

Be aware of processed foods – they are often filled with added sugar and starch – such as pre-made meatballs, various deli meats, and sausages. Also, note that fruits like apples, pears, and bananas contain a lot of carbohydrates.

"But they contain a lot of fiber and good vitamins" ... Yes they do, but they still count towards your carbohydrate intake. They contain a lot of fructose, which also raises our insulin levels, putting our body more easily into "storage mode."

If you absolutely can't do without fruit, choose a small handful of strawberries, raspberries, blueberries, or blackberries, and enjoy them with a good dollop of whipped cream.

For both strategies, it is essential to reduce (or completely avoid) carbohydrate- and starch-rich foods such as:

- Sugar, potatoes, rice, pasta, bread, and soda.

Instead, fill up on:

- Protein (e.g., beef, pork, chicken, fish, and eggs)
- Fat (e.g., real butter, cream, olive oil, avocado, and nuts)
- Vegetables (e.g., all kinds of cabbage, beans, cucumber, asparagus, and celery)

Chapter Five

THE GOOD FOODS

To get off to a good start, there are some foods I recommend you have in the house – this way, you can quickly make a healthy and delicious meal... even when you're in a hurry.

PROTEINS: MEAT, FISH, EGGS, AND PLANT-BASED SOURCES

Protein is an essential part of a Low Carb diet as it helps build and repair tissues, produces enzymes and hormones, and is an important energy source. Here are some of the best protein sources:

- **Meat:** Chicken, turkey, duck, beef, veal, pork, lamb, and game are excellent sources of protein. Don't shy away from eating the fat on the meat, the pork crackling on the roast, or the skin on the chicken.
- **Fish and Seafood:** Salmon, tuna, mackerel, herring, and other fatty fish are not only rich in protein, but also in omega-3 fatty acids, which are beneficial for

the heart. Shellfish like shrimp, crabs, and mussels are also good options.

- **Eggs:** Eggs are a versatile protein source that can be used for breakfast, lunch, and dinner. They are packed with essential amino acids and nutrients like vitamins B12 and D.
- **Plant-Based Sources:** For those who prefer plant-based proteins, tofu, tempeh, and edamame are good choices. These foods contain protein as well as fiber and other nutrients – be aware, however, that the carbohydrate count can add up quickly.

FATS: HEALTHY OILS, AVOCADO, NUTS, AND SEEDS

Healthy fats are crucial in a Low Carb diet, as they provide energy, support cell growth, and protect your organs. Choose high-quality fats and full-fat dairy products. Here are some of the best fat sources:

- **Healthy Oils:** Olive oil, coconut oil, and avocado oil are excellent sources of healthy fats. Use them for cooking, salad dressings, or as a topping.
- **Avocado:** Avocado is a fantastic source of monounsaturated fats, which are good for the heart. Use them in salads, smoothies, or as a simple snack with a little salt and pepper.

- **Olives:** Olives are low in carbohydrates and rich in healthy fats. They can be enjoyed as a snack or added to dishes.
- **Dairy Products:** Cream (38%), sour cream (38%), Greek yogurt (10%), and full-fat cheeses.
- **Nuts:** Almonds, walnuts, pecans, and macadamia nuts are low in carbohydrates and high in healthy fats and protein. They are perfect as snacks, or to add texture and flavor to your dishes.
- **Seeds:** Chia seeds, flaxseeds, sunflower seeds, and pumpkin seeds are rich in omega-3 fatty acids, fiber, and protein. They can be sprinkled on salads, yogurt, or mixed into smoothies.

VEGETABLES: THE BEST CHOICES FOR LOW CARB

Non-starchy vegetables are the cornerstone of a Low Carb diet. They are rich in vitamins, minerals, and fiber while being low in carbohydrates. Choose all vegetables that grow above ground. Here are some of the best choices:

- **Leafy Greens:** Spinach, kale, arugula, and lettuce are low in carbohydrates and high in nutrients. They can be used in salads, smoothies, or as a base for various dishes.
- **Cabbage:** Broccoli, cauliflower, cabbage, and brussels sprouts are excellent choices. They can be steam-

ed, roasted, or sautéed, and used as substitutes for potatoes, rice, and pasta.

- **Low-Carb Vegetables:** Zucchini, eggplant, bell peppers (green ones are lowest in carbs), cucumbers, and celery are versatile and can be used in many different dishes.
- **Mushrooms:** Mushrooms are also low in carbohydrates, and can add umami flavor to many dishes.

FRUITS: WHICH FRUITS ARE ALLOWED AND IN WHAT QUANTITIES

While fruit generally contains more sugar and carbohydrates than vegetables, there are still some low-carb options, you can enjoy in moderation:

- **Berries:** Strawberries, blueberries, raspberries, and blackberries are low in sugar and packed with antioxidants and fiber. A small handful of berries can be a great addition to yogurt or a salad.

By including the above good foods in your Low Carb diet, you can ensure you get a wide range of nutrients, while keeping your carbohydrate intake low. This can help you achieve your health and weight loss goals while enjoying delicious and satisfying meals.

Chapter Six

SNACKS AND MINI-MEALS

Snacks and mini-meals are not a necessity, as you often stay full between your main meals, but if the need arises, it's about choosing foods that keep you full and satisfied, while supporting your dietary goals. Here are some suggestions for quick and easy Low Carb snacks, ideas for mini-meals, and tips for managing sugar cravings.

QUICK AND EASY LOW CARB SNACKS

If hunger strikes between meals, it's important to have some easy and healthy Low Carb snacks ready. These snacks should be nutritious and easy to prepare. Here are some quick and easy suggestions:

- **Cheese and Nuts:** A combination of cheese and nuts provides a good balance of protein and healthy fats. Try eating cheddar cheese with almonds or walnuts.
- **Avocado with Lime and Salt:** Cut an avocado in

half, remove the pit, and drizzle with fresh lime juice and a sprinkle of salt. A filling and nutritious snack.

- **Hard-Boiled Eggs:** Hard-boiled eggs are perfect as a quick snack. They are packed with protein and healthy fats that keep you full longer.
- **Vegetable Sticks with Dip:** Cut vegetables like celery, cucumber, bell pepper, or carrots into sticks and serve them with a Low Carb dip like guacamole, cream cheese mixed with herbs and/or spices, or cauliflower hummus.
- **Olives:** A handful of olives is an easy snack that is low in carbohydrates and rich in healthy fats.

IDEAS FOR MINI-MEALS

Mini-meals can sometimes be necessary to keep your energy levels up and hunger at bay between larger meals. Here are some ideas for Low Carb mini-meals that are easy to prepare and take on the go:

- **Greek Yogurt with Berries and Nuts:** A portion of full-fat Greek yogurt topped with a handful of berries and chopped nuts provides a balanced mini-meal with protein, fat, and fiber.
- **Tuna Salad on Lettuce Leaves:** Mix tuna with may-

onnaise, chopped vegetables, and spices, and serve on crisp lettuce leaves for a light and tasty mini-meal.

- **Chicken Salad Wraps:** Use lettuce leaves as wraps and fill them with chicken salad made from cooked chicken, mayonnaise, celery, and spices.
- **Egg Muffins:** Make a batch of egg muffins with vegetables, cheese, and ham, and store them in the fridge for an easy snack or mini-meal.
- **Mixed Nuts and Seeds:** Make your own mix of nuts and seeds like almonds, walnuts, sunflower seeds, and pumpkin seeds.

HOW TO HANDLE SUGAR CRAVINGS

Sugar cravings can be a challenge, especially at the beginning of your Low Carb journey. Fortunately, there are several strategies you can use to handle any cravings:

- **Choose Low Carb Sweeteners:** Use natural sweeteners like stevia, erythritol, or monk fruit to satisfy your sweet tooth without increasing your carbohydrate intake. Try them in Low Carb baked goods or beverages.
- **Eat Regular Meals:** Stick to regular meals and mini-meals, to avoid long periods of hunger that can lead to cravings.

- **Drink Water:** Sometimes thirst can be mistaken for hunger. Make sure to drink plenty of water throughout the day – about 2.5 liters per day.
- **Healthy Alternatives:** When you crave something sweet, choose healthy alternatives like a handful of berries with whipped cream, a piece of dark chocolate (at least 70% cocoa), or a Low Carb dessert.
- **Distraction:** Find ways to distract yourself, when sugar cravings hit. Take a walk, read a book, or call a friend.

By having these snacks and mini-meals ready, as well as strategies to handle sugar cravings, you can more easily stick to your Low Carb diet, and thereby achieve your health and weight loss goals.

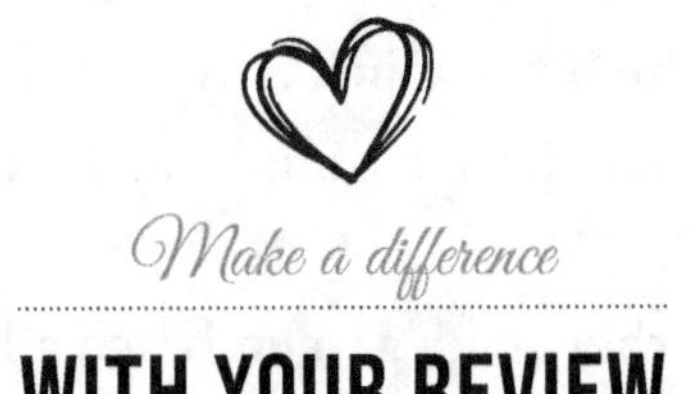

WITH YOUR REVIEW

Every journey to better health has its own unique path, and so does your experience with my "Beginner's Guide to Low Carb."

If you've started with this guide and explored the fundamentals of a Low Carb lifestyle, you now have valuable insights that can help others who are looking to achieve their weight loss goals, stabilize their blood sugar, and boost their energy levels.

Many individuals are in the same position you once were, eager to improve their health but uncertain about how to start. My aim with "Beginner's Guide to Low Carb" is clear: To make the transition to a Low Carb lifestyle as approachable and effective as possible for everyone.

This is where your voice becomes essential. While many consider a book by its title or cover, even more rely on reviews to guide their decisions.

So, for those looking to achieve their health goals, manage their weight, and feel more energized, I ask:

Could you take a moment to share your review?

Your review, which takes just a minute, could...

- help someone find a simple and effective path to weight loss.
- inspire another reader to embrace a healthier way of eating.
- guide someone in achieving stable blood sugar and more energy.
- assist others in overcoming the challenges of starting a new diet.
- motivate someone to make positive changes for their well being.

Ready to make a difference?

To do this, simply find the book on Amazon's website by scanning this QR code and locate the section to leave a review. Choose a star rating and write a couple of sentences.

With heartfelt thanks,
Rikke B. Eskildsen

P.S. If you think this guide could help others on their health journey, please share your knowledge of it with them. They'll appreciate it, and you might inspire them to make positive changes too!

Chapter Seven

KEEP IT SIMPLE

Eat until you're satisfied with meat, vegetables, and fats... eat when you're hungry and stop when you're full.

Weight loss doesn't have to be complicated, and you don't need pills, powders, or strange ingredients.

Avoid eating food that comes in colorful boxes and is labeled as "a healthy product"... because often it's not as healthy as the producers want you to think. As previously mentioned, a good rule of thumb is that food should contain a maximum of 5 grams of carbohydrates per 100 grams to avoid affecting our blood sugar too much.

By planning simple meals, using tips for quick and easy dishes, and preparing food in larger portions (batch cooking), you can also make the Low Carb lifestyle easier and less time-consuming. Here are some practical tips for keeping it simple.

HOW TO PLAN SIMPLE MEALS

Planning your meals in advance is key to keeping it simple and avoiding stress in daily life. Here are some steps to help you plan simple and nutritious Low Carb meals:

- **Make a Weekly Plan:** Start by planning your meals for a week at a time. Write down what you will eat for breakfast, lunch, and dinner each day. Include any snacks and mini-meals as well.
- **Choose Simple Recipes:** Stick to recipes with few ingredients and simple preparation methods. The fewer ingredients and steps, the easier it is to make the food.
- **Use the Same Ingredients for Multiple Days:** Plan meals that use the same ingredients in different ways. Chicken, broccoli, and avocado can e.g be used in a salad one day and in a stir-fry the next.
- **Prepare Ingredients in Advance:** Wash, chop, and store vegetables in advance, so they are ready to use. This saves time and makes it easier to prepare meals quickly.

TIPS FOR QUICK AND EASY DISHES

While it can be tempting to make complicated dishes, simple meals are often the best strategy in the long run.

Here are some tips for quick and easy Low Carb dishes:

- **One-Pan Meals:** Meals that can be prepared in one pan or pot save time on both cooking and cleanup. Try a one-pan chicken with vegetables or a quick stir-fry with beef and broccoli.
- **Salads:** Salads are versatile and quick to make. Use a base of leafy greens and add protein sources like chicken, tuna, or hard-boiled eggs. Top with healthy fats like avocado and nuts.
- **Oven Dishes:** Use the oven to make large portions of meat and vegetables at once. Make oven-baked salmon with asparagus or chicken breasts with broccoli and cauliflower.
- **Egg Dishes:** Eggs are a fantastic and quick protein source. Make a simple omelet with spinach and cheese, or try scrambled eggs with avocado and salsa.

PREPARATION AND BATCH COOKING

Preparation and batch cooking can save you time, and ensure that you always have healthy Low Carb meals ready to eat. Here are some tips to get started with batch cooking:

- **Plan Your Batch Cooking Days:** Choose one day a

week to spend a few hours cooking in larger portions. This could be Sunday or another day that suits you best.

- **Make Large Portions:** Prepare large portions of basic foods like meat, vegetables, and healthy fats. Divide them into smaller portions and store them in the fridge or freezer.
- **Use Airtight Containers:** Store your batch-cooked meals in airtight containers to keep them fresh. Label them with the date and contents for better organization.
- **Prepare Breakfast in Advance:** Make breakfast in portions that are easy to grab on the go. Try chia seed pudding, overnight oats (made with Low Carb ingredients), or egg muffins.
- **Freeze Extras:** Freeze extra portions of soups, stews, and oven dishes. This makes it easy to have healthy meals ready, when you're busy or don't feel like cooking.

By keeping your meals simple, using quick and easy recipes, and preparing food in larger portions, you can simplify your daily routine and ensure you always have healthy Low Carb meals ready.

Chapter Eight

ADAPT YOUR FAVORITE DISHES

One of the best ways to make the transition to a Low Carb lifestyle easier, is to start with your favorite dishes, and adapt them to fit your new dietary goals. By making Low Carb versions of classic dishes, family favorites, and festive meals, you can still enjoy the flavors and meals you love, and still prioritize your new lifestyle. Here are some tips for adapting different types of meals to a Low Carb version.

CLASSIC DISHES IN A LOW CARB VERSION

Many classic dishes can easily be adapted to a Low Carb version by replacing high-carbohydrate ingredients with lower carbohydrate alternatives. Here are some examples:

Spaghetti Bolognese: Replace spaghetti with zucchini noodles (zoodles) or spaghetti squash. Make your Bolognese sauce as usual with meat, tomatoes, and spices.

Pizza: Make a Low Carb pizza crust using cauliflower, almond flour, or use a ready-made Low Carb pizza crust.

Top with tomato sauce, cheese, and your favorite toppings.

Lasagna: Use slices of eggplant or zucchini instead of lasagna noodles or use thinly sliced turkey deli meat. Layer with meat sauce, ricotta, and mozzarella for a delicious Low Carb lasagna.

Fried Rice: Replace rice with finely chopped cauliflower to make a Low Carb version of fried rice. Add vegetables, eggs, and protein like chicken or shrimp.

FAMILY FAVORITES

Family favorites can often be adapted with minor adjustments. Here are some ideas:

Tacos: Use lettuce leaves or Low Carb tortillas instead of traditional tortillas. Fill with seasoned meat, avocado, cheese, salsa, and sour cream.

Burgers: Serve burgers without buns or use large lettuce leaves as wraps. Add all your favorite toppings like cheese, bacon, avocado, and sugar-free pickles.

Shepherd's Pie: Make the filling as usual with ground meat and vegetables, but replace the mashed potatoes with mashed cauliflower.

Chicken Nuggets: Make chicken nuggets by coating chicken pieces in almond flour or crushed pork rinds instead of breadcrumbs. Bake or fry until crispy and golden.

FESTIVE MEALS AND SPECIAL OCCASIONS

Even while eating Low Carb, you can still enjoy delicious festive meals and special occasions with some simple adjustments. Here are some suggestions:

Thanksgiving or Christmas Dinner: Serve turkey or ham with Low Carb sides like green beans, cauliflower mash, and a fresh green salad. Replace sugary desserts with Low Carb versions like pumpkin pie made with almond flour and erythritol.

BBQ Parties: Grill meats like steaks, chicken, or fish, and serve with grilled vegetables, a fresh salad, and Low Carb dips like guacamole or tzatziki.

Birthdays: Bake a Low Carb birthday cake using almond flour or coconut flour and sweeteners like stevia or erythritol. Decorate with whipped cream and berries for a festive and delicious dessert.

By transforming your favorite dishes into Low Carb versions, you can still savor the flavors and meals you love while sticking to your new dietary goals. The key is to be creative and find substitutions that align with your new lifestyle, ensuring you don't sacrifice taste or enjoyment.

Chapter Nine

EATING OUT ON A LOW CARB DIET

One of the challenges many people face, when following a Low Carb diet is dining out at restaurants. Fortunately, it is possible to enjoy meals out without compromising your new eating habits.

Here are some tips and strategies for navigating menus and making Low Carb choices, when eating out.

PREPARATION IS KEY

Before you go out to eat, it can be helpful to prepare a bit:

- **Check the Menu in Advance:** Many restaurants have their menus online. Look ahead of time to see which dishes best fit a Low Carb diet.
- **Plan Your Choices:** Decide in advance which dishes or ingredients to avoid, and what you can choose instead.

TIPS FOR EATING OUT

When you're at the restaurant, you can use these strategies to keep your meal Low Carb:

Ask for Modifications: Most restaurants are willing to accommodate special dietary needs. Ask if you can get vegetables instead of fries or a salad instead of bread.

Focus on Proteins and Vegetables: Choose dishes that mainly consist of proteins like meat, fish, or eggs, and ask for extra vegetables as a side.

Avoid Sugary Sauces and Dressings: Ask for sauces and dressings on the side, so you can control the amount. Choose olive oil and vinegar as a "safe" dressing.

Be Aware of Hidden Carbohydrates: Be cautious with soups and stews, as they often contain flour or sugar as thickening agents.

Asking for menu changes can be a bit daunting... but once you've done it a few times, it becomes easier and easier.

It's also a great feeling when you've stuck to your plan and have gained fantastic energy from your meal – unlike others who often need a nap or to "rest their stomachs."

EXAMPLES OF LOW CARB CHOICES

Here are some specific examples of how to choose Low Carb meals at different types of restaurants:

- **Steakhouse:** Choose a steak or grilled chicken with steamed vegetables or a salad. Avoid mashed potatoes and bread.
- **Italian Restaurant:** Order a grilled meat or fish dish and ask for extra vegetables instead of pasta. A Caprese salad with tomatoes, mozzarella, and basil is also a good choice.
- **Mexican Restaurant:** Choose a fajita salad without tortillas or a burrito bowl with meat, cheese, guacamole, and vegetables. Avoid rice and beans.
- **Asian Restaurant:** Choose dishes like grilled fish, chicken, or beef with vegetables. Ask for them without sugary sauces, and served with extra vegetables instead of rice or noodles.
- **Fast Food:** Many fast food chains now offer Low Carb options. Choose a burger without the bun, a salad with grilled chicken, or a wrap without tortillas.

BEVERAGES

Be mindful of your drink choices, when eating out:

- **Water:** Water with or without carbonation is always a "safe" choice.
- **Unsweetened Tea or Coffee:** These beverages are also good choices, but avoid sugar and sweetened creamers.
- **Low-Carb Alcohol:** If you choose to drink alcohol, opt for dry wines, champagne, or spirits like gin, vodka, or whiskey.

ENJOY THE MEAL

Eating out is also about enjoying the experience. By planning ahead and being mindful of your choices, you can still enjoy social gatherings and delicious meals without deviating from your Low Carb diet.

Remember, it's about balance, and an occasional indulgence won't ruin your progress as long as you quickly return to your healthy habits.

Chapter Ten

CHALLENGES IN TRANSITIONING TO FEWER CARBOHYDRATES

When you switch to a Low Carb diet, your body may go through a transition period, as it adapts to the new way of getting energy. This can result in some temporary challenges that are important to be aware of. By understanding these challenges and how to handle them, you can make the transition smoother and more enjoyable.

TRANSITION ISSUES: LOW CARB FLU

A common challenge in transitioning to fewer carbohydrates is what is often called "Low Carb Flu" or "Keto Flu." This is not an actual flu, but a set of symptoms that many experience in the first days or weeks of their Low Carb journey.

These symptoms occur because your body is adjusting from using carbohydrates as its primary energy source to burning fat. Here are some of the most common symptoms:

- Headache
- Fatigue
- Dizziness
- Irritability
- Mild muscle cramps
- Nausea

These symptoms are temporary and usually subside within a week or two as your body becomes better at burning fat for energy.

FLUID, ELECTROLYTES, AND SALT BALANCE

Another important factor to be aware of is that when you reduce your carbohydrate intake, your kidneys excrete more fluid and salt.

This can lead to dehydration and an electrolyte imbalance (e.g., sodium, potassium, and magnesium), which can worsen the symptoms of Low Carb flu.

When we reduce the amount of carbohydrates, the level of insulin in the body drops. Lower insulin levels cause the kidneys to excrete more sodium, which can lead to a lower sodium balance. This can result in symptoms like headaches, dizziness, and fatigue.

If our sodium levels drop, potassium can also fall, as these electrolytes are often seen together. Potassium is important for muscle function and heart rhythm, and a deficiency can lead to muscle cramps and weakness.

Many people do not get enough magnesium in their diet, and on a Low Carb diet this deficiency can become more pronounced. Magnesium is necessary for many biochemical reactions in the body, and a deficiency can result in muscle cramps, fatigue, and irritability.

Here are some tips to handle the above challenges:

- **Increase Your Water Intake:** Make sure to drink plenty of water to stay hydrated. This helps compensate for the increased fluid loss.
- **Potassium-Rich Foods:** Include potassium-rich foods like avocado, spinach, and nuts in your diet.
- **Magnesium Supplements:** Consider taking a magnesium supplement, especially if you experience muscle cramps or fatigue. Foods like green leafy vegetables, nuts, and seeds are also good sources of magnesium.
- **Increase Your Salt Intake:** Add extra salt to your

meals or drink a broth. This can help restore electrolyte balance and reduce symptoms like headaches and dizziness. Remembering to take in more salt is just as important as keeping the carbohydrates low – when we cook our food ourselves, we no longer get the same large amounts of salt from processed foods.

- **Electrolytes:** Consider taking electrolyte supplements that contain sodium, potassium, and magnesium to help maintain a healthy electrolyte balance – pay attention to the carbohydrate content and preferably choose some that are sweetened with stevia.

ENERGY AND FATIGUE

Initially, you might also experience a feeling of low energy and fatigue. This is because your body is not yet efficient at burning fat as fuel. Here are some ways to tackle this:

- **Eat Enough Fat:** Ensure you get enough healthy fats in your diet, as they are an important energy source on a Low Carb diet.
- **Eat Regularly:** Avoid long periods without food, especially in the beginning. Eat small meals and snacks regularly to keep your energy levels stable.
- **Exercise:** If you are used to regular exercise, you

might find that you don't have the same energy as before. But don't worry, the energy will return as your body gets used to using the new energy source.

- **Be Patient:** Remember that these symptoms are temporary. Your body will gradually adapt and start burning fat more efficiently, resulting in more stable energy levels.

LONG-TERM ADAPTATION

Once your body has adapted to the new diet, you will likely experience increased energy, stable blood sugar levels, and improved mental clarity. For many people, these benefits are worth going through the short-term adjustment period.

If you experience persistent or severe symptoms, it's important to consult a doctor or a nutritionist to ensure that your Low Carb diet is balanced and appropriate for your individual needs.

By being aware of these challenges and taking steps to manage them, you can make the transition to a Low Carb lifestyle easier and more successful.

Chapter Eleven

HELP AND GUIDANCE

When starting a Low Carb journey, many questions and doubts can arise. It is important to have access to reliable information and support to ensure that you get the most out of your new lifestyle. In this section, I will address some of the most common questions, clarify myths and misconceptions about Low Carb, and give you tips to stay motivated.

FREQUENTLY ASKED QUESTIONS

What is a Low Carb Diet?

A Low Carb diet involves reducing the intake of carbo-hydrates, and replacing them with proteins and healthy fats. This helps stabilize blood sugar levels and promotes weight loss.

How Many Carbohydrates Should I Consume Daily?

It varies from person to person, but many Low Carb diets recommend staying under 50 grams of net carbohydrates per day. Some more restrictive versions, like the ketogenic diet, may require less than 20 grams.

Is it Safe to Eat Few Carbohydrates?

For most people, a Low Carb diet is safe and can have many health benefits. However, it is important to talk to a doctor, especially if you have existing medical conditions. For example, if you are on diabetes medication that lowers your blood sugar, it is important to have your doctor on board to adjust the medication as needed, due to the lower carbohydrate intake in your diet. Be extra careful if you take insulin, as you risk having too low blood sugar, when combining it with a Low Carb diet.

Will I Feel Fatigued or Unwell Initially?

Some people experience fatigue and other symptoms in the beginning, known as "Low Carb flu." This is due to the body's adjustment to a lower carbohydrate intake, and the symptoms usually disappear after a few days.

MYTHS AND MISCONCEPTIONS ABOUT LOW CARB

Myth: Low Carb Means No Carbohydrates at All

Truth: A Low Carb diet reduces, but does not necessarily eliminate carbohydrates. The focus is on choosing carbohydrates from non-starchy vegetables and berries.

Myth: Low Carb Diet is Not Balanced

Truth: A well-planned Low Carb diet includes a variety of foods that provide all necessary nutrients. It's about choosing quality foods like vegetables, healthy fats, and proteins.

Myth: You Can't Get Enough Fiber on a Low Carb Diet

Truth: Many non-starchy vegetables are high in fiber and low in carbohydrates, making it possible to get sufficient fiber.

Myth: Low Carb Diets Are Only for Weight Loss

Truth: Besides weight loss, Low Carb diets can help improve blood sugar levels, increase energy levels, and support overall health.

TIPS TO STAY MOTIVATED

Here are some tips to keep you motivated:

- **Set Realistic Goals:** Start with small, achievable goals and celebrate your progress. This can help keep you motivated and make the process less overwhelming.

- **Stay Informed:** Read books, articles, and studies about Low Carb diets to understand the health benefits, and how to best follow the diet.

- **Find Support:** Join online communities or local groups with others, who follow a Low Carb lifestyle. Sharing experiences and getting support can be invaluable.

- **Plan Your Meals:** Plan your meals and snacks in advance to avoid temptations, and ensure you always have healthy options available.
- **Experiment with Recipes:** Try new recipes and ingredients to keep your meals interesting and varied. This can help avoid boredom and keep you engaged in your diet.
- **Be Patient:** Weight loss and health improvements take time. Be patient with yourself and remember that persistence is key to long-term results.

Remember, everyone's journey is unique, and the most important thing is to find a balance that works for you.

Chapter Twelve

RECIPES FOR INSPIRATION

Having a range of tasty and easy recipes on hand can make it much easier to follow a Low Carb diet. On the next pages, I have gathered some inspiration for you and created a meal plan for 1 week with suggestions for breakfast, lunch, and dinner.

Feel free to swap the meals around to suit you best, and if you're the type who doesn't eat breakfast, just skip it – or delay it until you're hungry. Even though I've written breakfast, lunch, and dinner, you're also welcome to eat dinner recipes for breakfast – sometimes it can actually be an advantage, as it keeps you full longer... just adjust it to fit your needs.

Make extra portions if needed, so you have easy meals for a later time – most dishes can be easily frozen.

Also feel free to substitute ingredients if you have something else on hand that can be used. Don't be afraid to experiment a bit – the key is to keep things simple and to adjust the recipes to suit your tastes.

It is very important that you find what works for you and what you enjoy eating. Whether it's swapping out vegetables, using a different type of protein, or adjusting seasonings, adapt the recipes to make them your own. The flexibility to make changes will help you stay engaged with your Low Carb journey and make it more enjoyable.

Switching to a Low Carb lifestyle can be an exciting journey towards better health and well-being. With the right tools, knowledge, and inspiration, you are well-equipped to take control of your diet and achieve your goals. Remember, success with a Low Carb diet is about finding a balance that fits you and your lifestyle.

Whether you're looking for weight loss, stable blood sugar, or increased energy, Low Carb can be the way forward. Take it one step at a time, be patient with yourself, and enjoy the process.

Enjoy and bon appétit!

MEAL PLAN

Meal suggestions for 1 week

Scan the QR-code to download printable Meal Plan, Recipes and list of The Good Foods.

Feel free to swap the order around to fit your schedule.

	Breakfast	*Lunch*	*Dinner*
MONDAY	Eggs with mayo and shrimp **(page 56)**	Chicken salad on lettuce leaves **(page 61)**	Meat sauce with vegetables **(page 68)**
THUESDAY	Greek yogurt with nuts and berries **(page 57)**	Egg salad on lettuce leaves **(page 62)**	Sausage stew with cauliflower rice **(page 69)**
WEDENSDAY	Scrambled eggs with sausages **(page 60)**	Tomato salad with mozzarella **(page 63)**	Oven-baked salmon with sesame **(page 70)**
THURSDAY	Smoked salmon with cottage cheese **(page 58)**	Egg and tuna salad on lettuce leaves **(page 64)**	Chicken curry with cauliflower rice **(page 71)**
FRIDAY	Greek yogurt with nuts and berries **(page 57)**	Parma ham with cream cheese **(page 65)**	Fried pork belly with parsley sauce **(page 72)**
SATURDAY	Cinnamon omelet with crème fraîche **(page 59)**	Chicken drum sticks with tzatziki **(page 66)**	Fathead pizza with salad **(page 73)**
SUNDAY	Scrambled eggs with bacon **(page 60)**	Chaffle with chicken and bacon **(page 67)**	Steak with beans and béarnaise mayo **(page 74)**

EGGS WITH MAYO AND SHRIMP

1 serving

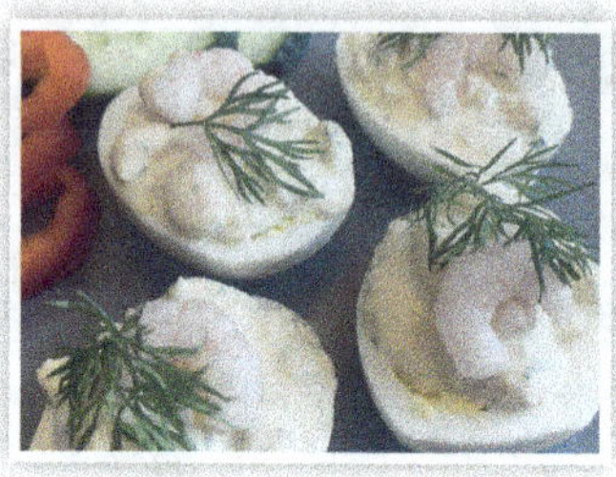

3 eggs
2 tbsp mayonnaise
2 tbsp crème fraîche 38%
1.8 oz / 50 g shrimp (chopped into smaller pieces)
1/4 tsp cumin
1/2 tbsp dill
Lemon juice, salt, and pepper

Boil the eggs for 8-10 minutes and let them cool. Mix mayonnaise and crème fraîche with spices, a bit of lemon juice, and dill. Cut the eggs in half and remove the yolks, which you chop and mix into the dressing along with the chopped shrimp.

Put the filling back into the halved eggs and garnish with a bit of dill if desired.

Serve with some vegetables if desired.

GREEK YOGURT WITH NUTS AND BERRIES

1 serving

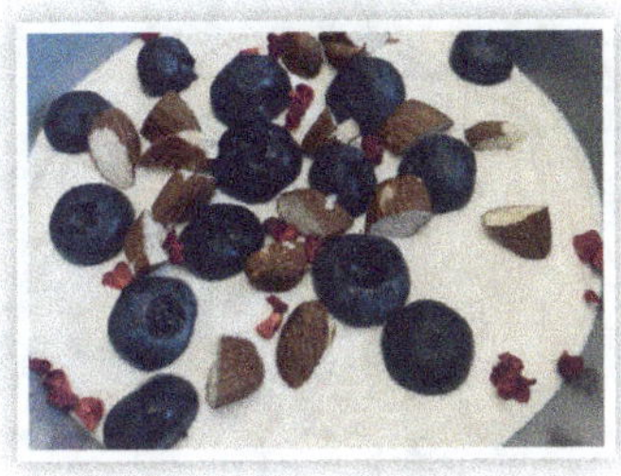

3/4 cup / 200 g Greek yogurt 10%
2-3 tbsp heavy cream 38%
Optional: a bit of vanilla powder
Some mixed nuts (e.g., almonds, hazelnuts, or walnuts)

Mix the Greek yogurt with heavy cream and vanilla powder, and sprinkle with chopped nuts.

Optionally, you can also sprinkle with some blueberries or raspberries.
You can also make a compote with rhubarb, lemon juice, vanilla seeds, and a bit of sweetener, which you boil in a small pot.

SMOKED SALMON WITH COTTAGE CHEESE

1 serving

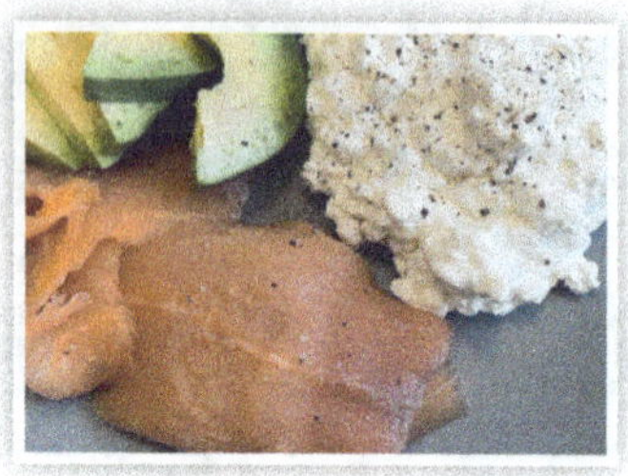

1.8 oz / 50 g smoked salmon
1/2 cup / 100 g cottage cheese 4%
1 avocado
Salt and pepper

Remove the pit, slice the avocado, and arrange it on a plate with the cottage cheese and salmon.

CINNAMON OMELET WITH CRÈME FRAÎCHE

1 serving

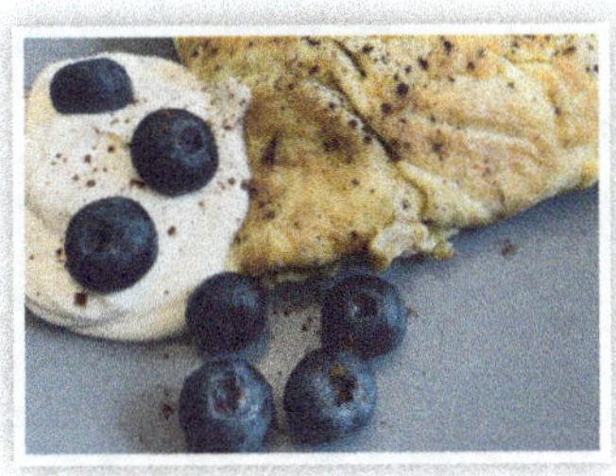

2-3 eggs
2-3 tbsp heavy cream 38%
1/2 tbsp cinnamon
1 large tbsp crème fraîche 38% or whipped cream
1 large tbsp butter for frying

Whisk eggs, heavy cream, and cinnamon together in a bowl.
Melt the butter in a pan and cook the egg mixture until it is set.
Serve with a good dollop of crème fraîche or whipped cream.

You can also try varying it with other spices such as vanilla, cocoa,
or cardamom.

SCRAMBLED EGGS WITH SAUSAGES/BACON

1 serving

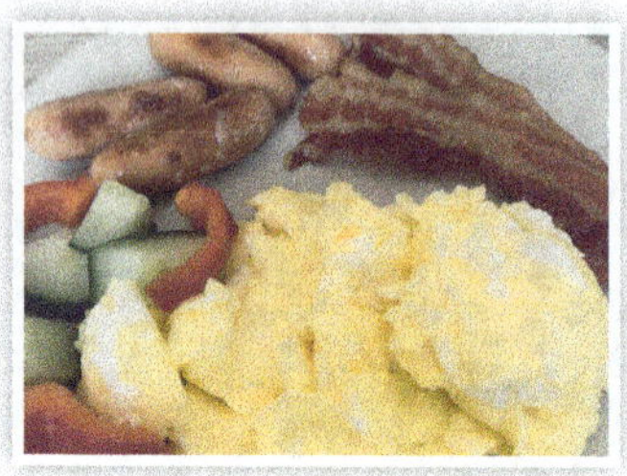

2-3 eggs
2-3 tbsp heavy cream 38%
Salt and pepper
1 tbsp butter or coconut oil for frying

Whisk the eggs together in a bowl with the heavy cream, and add a bit of salt and pepper. Heat the pan and cook the eggs in butter or coconut oil. Stir the egg mixture until it is set.

Serve with some fried sausages (about 100 g) or bacon (3-4 slices) if desired. You can also enjoy it with some cucumber slices, bell pepper, and tomato.

CHICKEN SALAD ON LETTUCE LEAVES

1 serving

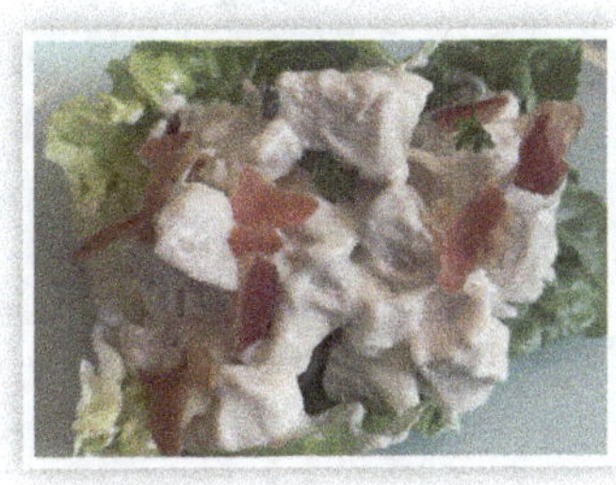

1-3 romaine lettuce leaves

3.5 oz / 100 g cooked chicken

1-2 slices fried bacon

0.9 oz / 25 g white asparagus

0.9 oz / 25 g mushrooms

Butter for frying

1.5 tbsp mayonnaise

1.5 tbsp crème fraîche 38%

1/4 tsp Dijon mustard

A pinch of curry powder (optional)

Salt and pepper

Fry the mushrooms in butter and let them cool on a piece of paper towel.

Mix the dressing by combining mayonnaise, crème fraîche, mustard, and spices.

Cut the chicken into cubes and the asparagus into smaller pieces, then mix them with the dressing.

Serve in romaine lettuce leaves, sprinkling the bacon pieces on top.

EGG SALAD ON LETTUCE LEAVES

1 serving

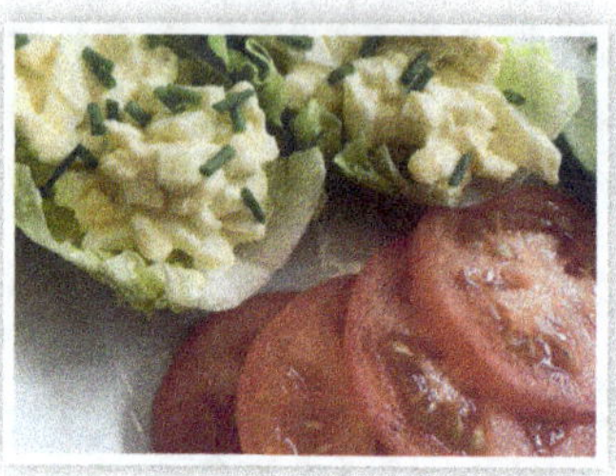

1-3 romaine lettuce leaves
2-3 eggs
2-3 tbsp mayonnaise
1/2 tbsp curry powder
Salt and pepper

Boil the eggs for 8-10 minutes and then let them cool.
Chop the eggs (you can use an egg slicer) and mix them first with the curry powder and a bit of salt and pepper. Finally, mix in the mayonnaise.

Serve in romaine lettuce leaves. Garnish with cress or chives if desired, and eat with some extra vegetables if you like.

TOMATO SALAD WITH MOZZARELLA

1 serving

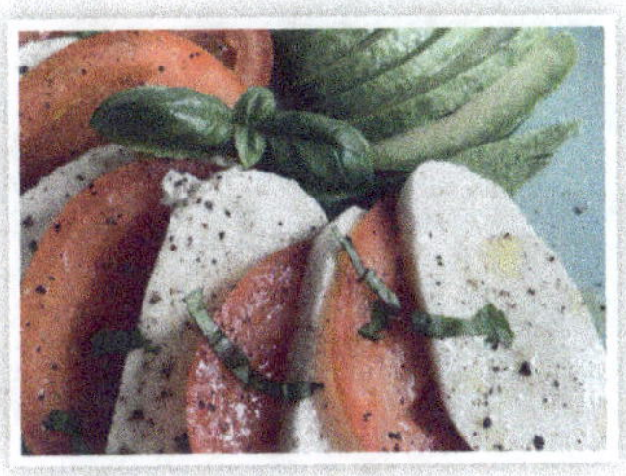

4.4 oz / 125 g fresh mozzarella (1 ball)

1-2 tomatoes

1-2 tbsp olive oil

Basil

1 avocado

Salt and pepper

Slice the mozzarella and tomato, and arrange them on a plate by alternating slices of mozzarella and tomato.
Drizzle with olive oil and sprinkle with salt, pepper, and fresh basil.

Serve with 1 sliced avocado if desired.

EGG AND TUNA SALAD

1 serving

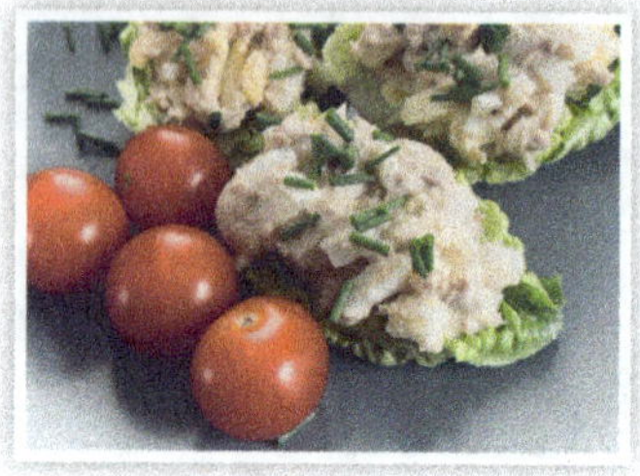

1 can of tuna (in water)

1 egg

3 tbsp mayonnaise

A bit of lemon juice

Salt and pepper

Boil the egg for 8-10 minutes and then let it cool.
Mash the tuna with a fork. Chop the egg (you can use an egg slicer) and mix it with the tuna and mayonnaise. Season with lemon juice, salt, and pepper.

Serve in romaine lettuce leaves. Garnish with cress or chives if desired, and eat with some extra vegetables if you like.

PARMA HAM WITH CREAM CHEESE

1 serving

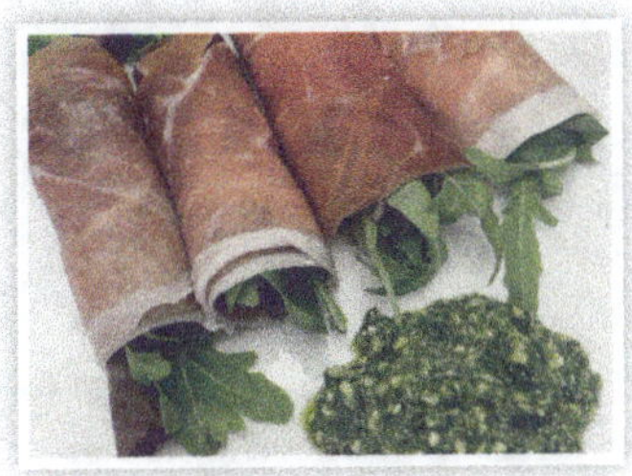

2.8 oz / 80 g Parma ham
1.8 oz / 50 g plain cream cheese (not light)
1 tbsp chopped parsley
1 handful mixed salad leaves
– optionally arugula Salt and pepper

Mix the cream cheese with the chopped parsley and season with salt and pepper. Lay the slices of Parma ham on a cutting board and distribute dollops of cream cheese on each slice.

Then, add the salad leaves and roll the Parma ham around the filling into small rolls.

Serve with a couple of tablespoons of green pesto if desired.

CHICKEN DRUM STICKS WITH TZATZIKI

1 serving

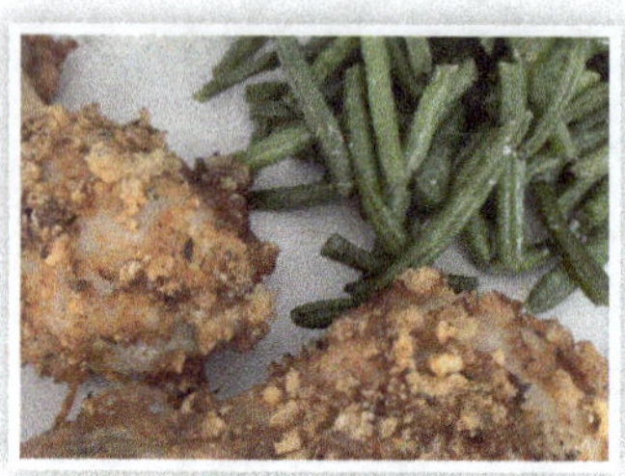

2-3 chicken drum sticks

1 egg

1.8 oz / 50 g crushed pork rinds

Optional: grill seasoning or paprika

2 cups / 200 g green beans

1 tbsp melted butter

Tzatziki

1/2 cup / 100 g Greek yogurt 10%

1/2 cucumber

1 small clove garlic (pressed)

Salt and pepper

Crush pork rinds (without fat edge) in a mini chopper and mix them with grill seasoning or paprika. Dip the chicken legs in beaten egg and then in the crushed pork rinds. Place them on a baking sheet with parchment paper and bake in the oven at 375°F / 190°C for 35-40 minutes (until the chicken is cooked).

Toss the green beans in melted butter and sprinkle with salt – bake them in the oven along with the chicken the last 20 minutes.

Grate the cucumber and squeeze out the excess water. Mix with Greek yogurt, garlic, salt, and pepper.

Optionally, you can cook the chicken as you usually do.

CHAFFLE WITH CHICKEN AND BACON

1 serving

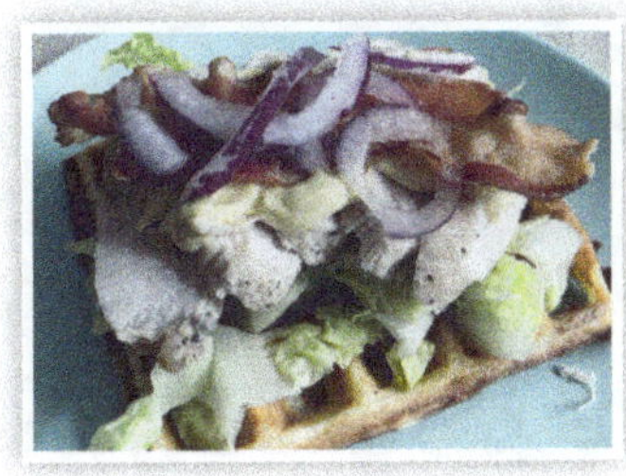

Chaffle:

2 eggs

1 cup / 1-2 dl grated mozzarella

Salt and pepper

1.8 oz / 50 g cooked chicken

1-2 slices fried bacon

A bit of salad and red onion

Curry dressing:

3.5 tbsp mayonnaise

3.5 tbsp crème fraîche 38%

1/2 tsp apple cider vinegar

1 tsp curry powder

1/2 tsp Sukrin Gold

Salt, pepper, and a bit of turmeric

Mix the eggs and grated cheese together and season with a bit of salt and pepper. Then cook the chaffles in a waffle iron.

Mix the dressing and use 1-2 tablespoons – save the rest for later. Sukrin Gold can be replaced with your prefered sweetener if desired. Arrange the chaffles with salad, chicken, dressing, bacon, and a bit of red onion.

MEAT SAUCE WITH VEGETABLES

4 servings

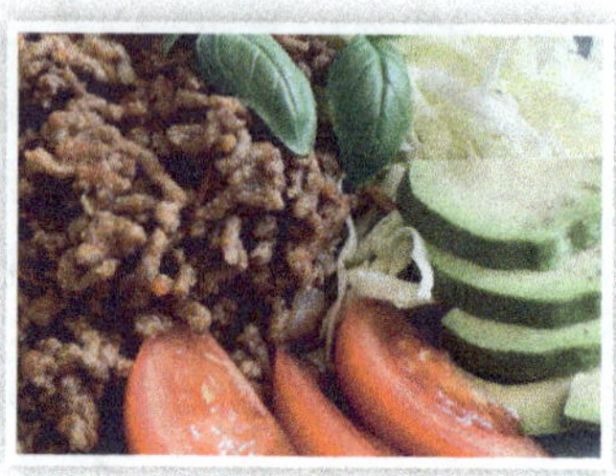

1.3 lbs / 600 g ground meat
1 red bell pepper
10 mushrooms
1 onion

1-2 cloves garlic
1 tbsp tomato paste
1 can chopped tomatoes
Salt and pepper

Clean the bell pepper and mushrooms, and cut them into smaller pieces. Peel and chop the onion and garlic, and sauté them in butter in a pan.

Add the ground meat and cook until browned and fully cooked.

Next, add the tomato paste, mushrooms, and bell pepper, and cook for a few minutes. Finally, add the chopped tomatoes, salt, and pepper.

Let the dish simmer for about 10 minutes and adjust seasoning with more salt and pepper if needed.

Serve with finely shredded cabbage as a substitute for traditional pasta. You can also sauté some sliced zucchini or make a delicious salad.

SAUSAGE STEW WITH CAULIFLOWER RICE

4 servings

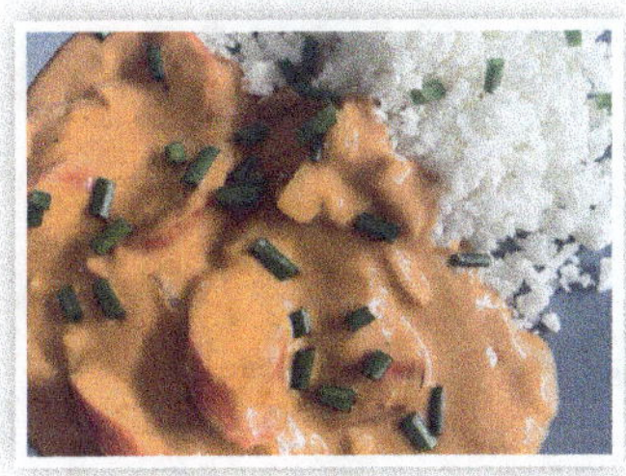

1.3 lbs / 600 g sausage (with a high meat content of over 70%)

1 onion	1 tsp Dijon mustard
3 tbsp tomato paste	1 tbsp paprika
1 cup / 2.5 dl heavy cream 38%	1 tsp salt
1 cup / 2.5 dl crème fraîche 38%	A bit of pepper
2 tbsp veal stock	2 tbsp butter for frying

Slice the sausages. Peel and finely chop the onion.

Melt the butter and sauté the sausages, onion, and tomato paste. Then add the heavy cream, crème fraîche, stock, mustard, and paprika. Season with salt and pepper and let it simmer until the sauce reaches a nice consistency.

Optionally, serve with cauliflower rice: Grate a cauliflower and sauté it in butter in a pan. Season with salt.

OVEN-BAKED SALMON WITH SESAME

2 servings

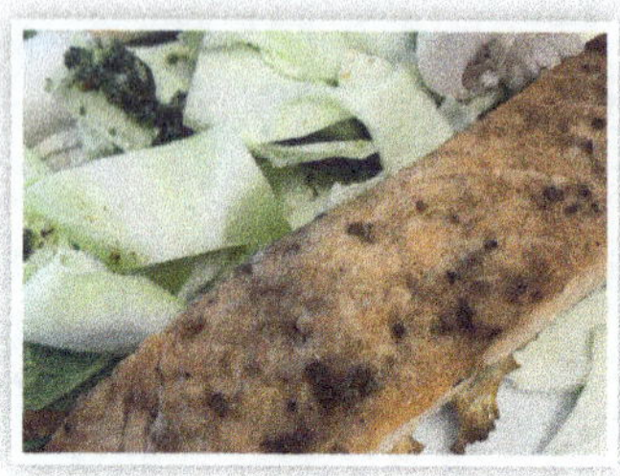

2 pieces of fresh salmon
 (about 8.8 oz / 250 g each)
1/2 lemon, sliced

Marinade:
2 tbsp oregano
1 tsp ground cumin

1/2 tsp ground chili
1/2 tsp salt
3 tbsp olive oil
2 tbsp soy sauce
2 tbsp sesame seeds

Preheat the oven to 340°C / 170°C.
Place the salmon pieces in an ovenproof dish and mix the marinade ingredients in a bowl.
Pour the marinade over the salmon and sprinkle with extra sesame seeds if desired. Arrange some lemon slices around the salmon and place the dish in the oven.
Bake for about 15 minutes.

Serve with a good salad.

CHICKEN CURRY WITH CAULIFLOWER RICE

4 servings

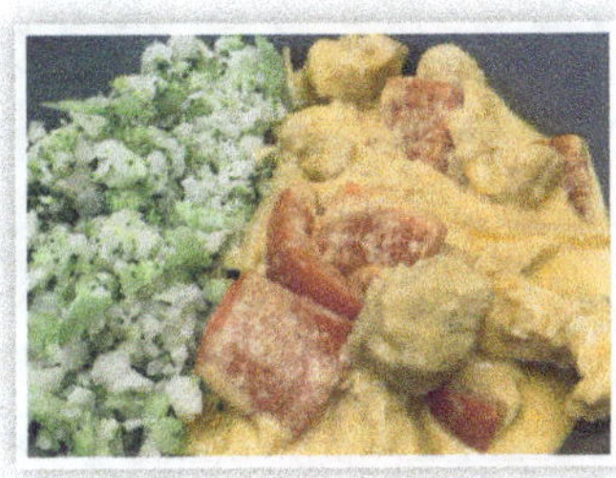

1.3 lbs / 600 g chicken breast	2 cups / 5 dl heavy cream 38%
1 onion	0.85 cup / 2 dl crème fraîche 38%
1-2 red bell peppers	2 tbsp soy sauce
2-3 tbsp curry powder	Salt and pepper
1 tbsp paprika	3 tbsp butter for frying

Cut the chicken breasts into pieces and fry them in the butter in a large pot.

Wash and chop the bell peppers. Peel and cut the onion into wedges.

When the chicken is nearly cooked through, add the bell peppers, onion, curry powder, and paprika. Sauté for about 3 minutes.

Then add the heavy cream, crème fraîche, soy sauce, and pepper – and season with salt to taste.

Serve with broccoli or cauliflower rice **(see page 69).**

FRIED PORK BELLY WITH PARSLEY SAUCE

4 servings

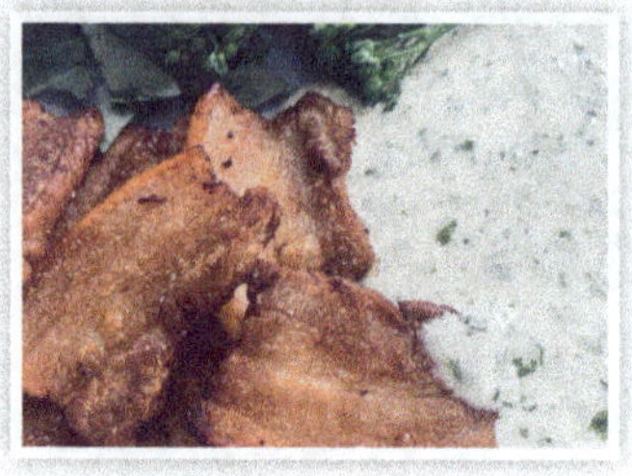

1.8 lbs / 800 g pork belly slices
Salt and pepper

Parsley Sauce:
2 tbsp butter
2 tbsp plain cream cheese
1.25 cups / 3 dl heavy cream
1 small bunch of parsley

Salt the pork belly slices well and cook them using your preferred method (pan-fry, bake, grill, etc.).

Melt the butter in a saucepan and add the cream. Let the cream come to a simmer over low heat, then add the cream cheese. Once the sauce has reached the desired consistency, add the chopped parsley and season with salt and pepper.

Serve with lightly cooked broccoli or cauliflower.

FATHEAD PIZZA

1 serving

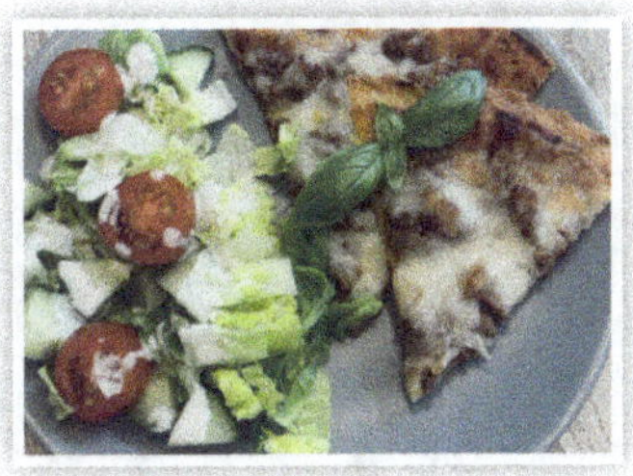

5 oz / 140 g shredded mozzarella

2-3 tbsp psyllium husk or almond flour

1 egg

1 cup / 2.5 dl tomato passata

3 tbsp grated Parmesan

2 tbsp Sukrin Gold

1.5 tsp oregano

0.5 tsp basil

1 tsp garlic powder

0.75 tsp onion powder

0.25 tsp ground black pepper

Toppings: For example, leftover meat sauce.
Or ham, mushrooms, onion, and bell pepper. Or pepperoni.

Melt mozzarella in a saucepan. Then add an egg and the psyllium husk or almond flour and mix well. Roll out the dough between two pieces of parchment paper. Prick the dough with a fork and bake the crust for about 10 minutes at 375°F / 190°C – until it is slightly colored. Remove the pizza crust from the oven, spread it with some of the pizza sauce, and then add your preferred toppings. Sprinkle with a bit more shredded cheese dind put the pizza back in the oven until the cheese is melted. Serve the pizza with a good salad.

STEAK WITH BEANS AND BEARNAISE MAYO

1 serving

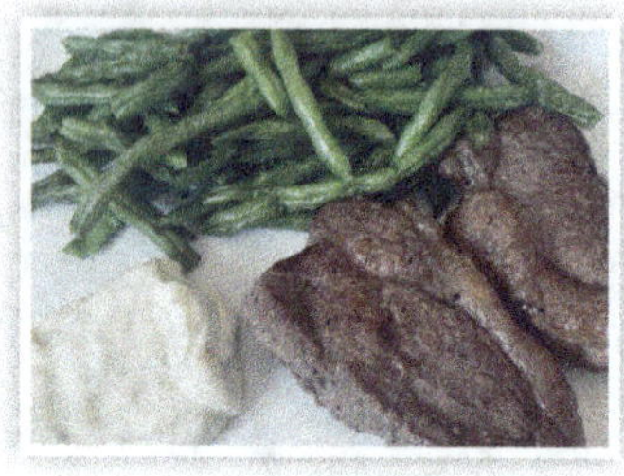

5.3 oz / 150 g steak

2 cups / 200 g green beans
1 tbsp butter
2-3 tbsp mayonnaise
Béarnaise essence
Tarragon
Salt and pepper

Toss the green beans in melted butter and sprinkle with salt – bake them in the oven at 375°F / 190°C for about 20 minutes.

Béarnaise mayo: Mix the mayonnaise with a few drops of Béarnaise essence, a small pinch of tarragon, and a bit of salt.

Cook the steak in butter in a pan for 2-4 minutes on each side (depending on how well-done you like it).

Season with salt and pepper and serve everything on a plate.

RESOURCES

Dr. David Unwin, MD, is an award-winning general practitioner (or family doctor) known for pioneering the low-carb approach in the UK. Through the years, Dr. Unwin has been highly recognized for his work within his field.

In 2015, Dr. Unwin was made a UK Royal College of General Practitioners expert clinical advisor for his dedicated efforts within the areas of patient communication and type 2 diabetes.
www.phcuk.org/sugar

—

DietDoctor — founded by Dr. Andreas Eenfeldt, MD, in 2011, after starting up in Sweden in 2007.

Their guides are written and reviewed by medical doctors and experts, based on scientific evidence and trusted by practicing physicians.

To stay unbiased they show no ads, they sell no products and they take no money from industry. Their website does not host any form of advertisements.
www.dietdoctor.com